NATURAL ARTHRITIS TREATMENT

DR MIRIAM KINAI

ISBN: 1490488855

ISBN-13: 978-1490488851

CONTENTS

ACKNOWLEDGMENTS

I would like to express my sincere gratitude to everyone who contributed in one way or another to the development of this publication.

I would especially like to thank http://www.zazzle.com/ChristianArtGifts for their photographs.

1

DIET THERAPY

Dietary modifications that you can help relieve joint pains include:

1.

Eat fresh pineapples

Pineapples contain bromelain which is an enzyme that helps reduce inflammation. Therefore eat fresh pineapples regularly since freezing and caning them destroys this enzyme.

***

2.

Eat cherries

Cherries contain natural anti-inflammatory properties that can reduce joint pain and damage. Therefore, eat 12 cherries each day to manage arthritis.

***

3.

Eat more antioxidant rich foods

Increase your intake of antioxidant rich foods like carrots, dark green leafy vegetables, sweet potatoes and citrus fruits like oranges and lemons. This is because antioxidants like vitamin A, C, E and selenium help reduce the inflammation in the joints.

***

4.

Eat more fatty fish

Increase your intake of fatty fish like salmon and tuna which provide omega 3 fatty acids since these have been shown to decrease joint pain and morning stiffness.

***

5.

Add flaxseed oil

Flaxseed oil provides another type of anti-inflammatory fatty acids which are also important for joint mobility. Therefore take 1 tablespoon of flaxseed oil each day to get adequate amounts of omega 3 fatty acids. You can add it to your salads or smoothies.

***

6.

Eat more calcium rich foods

Increase your intake of calcium and vitamin D from milk, yoghurt, cheese and other dairy products since these are vital for bone health.

***

7.

Avoid trans fats

Reduce your consumption of trans fats (trans fatty acids) by avoiding margarine, vegetable shortening and processed foods cakes and cookies and fast foods like French fries and doughnuts.

* * * * *

2

SUPPLEMENTS

Supplements that are used for natural arthritis treatment include:

1.

Glucosamine sulfate

This is a natural constituent of healthy cartilage that may help rebuild cartilage and slow the progression of the disease. It can be taken at a dose of 750 mg twice a day.

2.

Chondroitin sulphate

Chondroitin sulphate is an effective supplement for arthritis since it helps repair and maintain cartilage and connective tissue. It is usually taken at a dose of 400 mg three times a day.

***

3.

Methylsulfonylmethane (MSM)

Methysulfonylmethane (MSM) 2-3 grams per day is also taken to treat arthritis.

***

4.

SAM-e

S-adenosylmethionine has been shown to reduce arthritic joint pain and it was found to have pain reducing effects that were comparable to those of ibuprofen which is an anti-inflammatory drug. It can be taken at doses of 400 mg daily.

***

5.

Omega 3 fatty acids

Consider taking fish oil supplements with omega 3 fatty acids since they have been shown to decrease joint pain and morning stiffness. Omega fatty acids can be taken at doses of 2,000 mg three times a day.

***

6.

A daily multi-vitamin

Take a multi-vitamin, multi-mineral supplement that contains:

a. Vitamin C which is needed for collagen repair

b. Calcium and vitamin D which are crucial for bone health

* * * * *

3

HERBS

Herbs that are used to manage arthritis include:

1.

Boswelia or Frankincense

Boswelia or Frankincense is a natural anti-inflammatory which is useful for preventing joint damage and reducing joint pain.

It's anti-inflammatory action has been proven to reduce joint pain. It can be taken at a dose of 900 mg a day.

***

2.

Willow Bark

Willow bark, which produces natural aspirin, is another natural anti-inflammatory that can reduce joint pain and damage without causing the gastritis and ulcers that are associated with prescription analgesics.

Studies have shown that it is twice as effective as analgesic like Motrin and Vioxx.

3.

Ginger

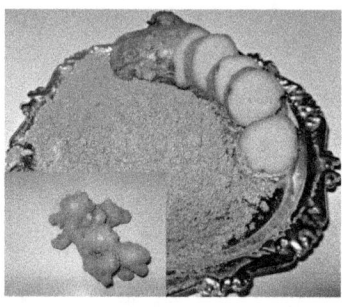

Ginger has anti-inflammatory properties which reduce the pain of arthritis. A study done in Miami revealed that ginger was effective in relieving the pain of patients with osteoarthritis.

Ginger is thought to decrease the pain of arthritis by increasing blood supply and also because of its anti-inflammatory properties.

Therefore, take half a teaspoon of ginger powder or 30 grams of fresh ginger each day. Keep in mind that these are more pronounced when ginger is used with turmeric to reduce the pain and swelling of arthritis.

4.

Turmeric

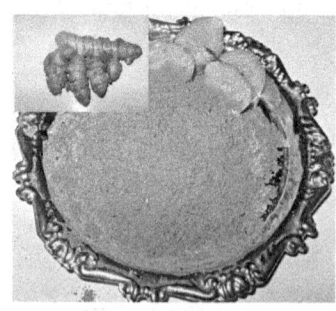

Turmeric contains curcumin which has anti-inflammatory properties and is useful for reliving the pain and swelling of arthritis. These effects are also beneficial for the management of carpal tunnel syndrome.

Turmeric enhances the effects of ginger when they are both used to treat arthritis.

***

5.

Feverfew

Feverfew (Tanacetum parthenium) has anti-inflammatory effects which are useful for the management of arthritis. It can be taken at a dose of one capsule twice a day.

6.

Capsaicin

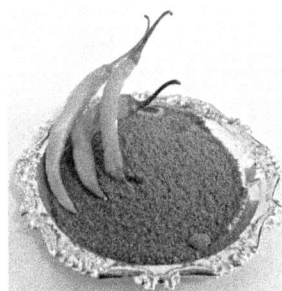

Cayenne pepper contains capsaicin which has pain relieving effects and is useful for the management of pain from rheumatoid arthritis and osteoarthritis. This capsaicin first stimulates the nerves and then decreases the intensity of the pain stimuli or signal. It is usually applied as a 0.025% capsaicin cream to treat arthritis pain four times a day.

* * * * *

4

ESSENTIAL OILS

Aromatherapy is the use of essential oils for their healing benefits. Essential oils that are used to manage arthritis include lavender, eucalyptus and Roman chamomile.

Lavender Essential Oil

Botanical name: Lavendula officinalis

Perfumery Note: Middle note

Lavender Essential Oil Safety Information

1. Do not use it in pregnancy especially the first 3 months.

2. Do not use it if you are breastfeeding.

3. Do not use it on young children as it may cause breast development in boys (gynaecomastia) and girls (pre-pubescent breast development).

4. Avoid it if you have low blood pressure as you may feel drowsy.

***

Eucalyptus Essential Oil

Name: Eucalyptus globulus

Perfumery Note: Top note

Eucalyptus Essential Oil Safety Information

1. Do not ingest it as it can be fatal when taken orally.

2. Do not use it if you have epilepsy.

3. Do not use it if you have high blood pressure.

4. Do not apply it near a baby's nostrils.

5. Do not store it near homeopathic formulas as it may affect them.

***

Roman Chamomile Essential Oil

Name: Chamaemelum nobile

Perfumery Note: Middle note

Roman Chamomile Essential Oil Safety Information

1. Avoid using it in pregnancy.

2. Avoid using it if you are allergic to ragweed, asters, chrysanthemums and asters.

3. Avoid it if you have asthma.

***

Using Essential Oils for Arthritis Treatment

The first step in using essential oils is to do a patch test on each of the essential oils that you want to use.

To do this, simply apply the essential oil that has been diluted with a carrier oil on the inner aspect of your elbow, bandage it and wait for 24 hours to see if you will develop rashes or swelling or any other sign of an allergic reaction. If you do, do not use that essential oil.

The second step is to create the essential oil blend that you will use. A simple "Arthritis Treatment Blend" can be made by mixing 20 drops of Lavender essential oil, 20 drops of Roman chamomile essential oil and 30 drops of Eucalyptus essential oil in a dark bottle.

We will refer to this mixture as the "Arthritis Treatment Blend" in our recipes. Therefore, if the recipe says, "Add 12 drops of Arthritis Treatment Blend", you simply add 12 drops of this mixture.

If you just want to buy one aromatherapy oil to experiment with, I would recommend eucalyptus essential oil. Likewise, if the recipe says, "Add 12 drops of Arthritis Treatment Blend", you simply add 12 drops of eucalyptus essential oil.

Aromatherapy Bath.

Create a relaxing bath by dispersing 12 drops of the "Arthritis Treatment Blend" in your warm bath water. You can also mix it with milk to help it disperse. Soaking in this warm bath especially in the morning can relax stiff joints and provide arthritis pain relief.

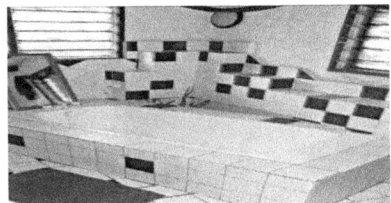

Bath Gel.

Add 50 drops (2.5 ml or ½ teaspoons) of the "Arthritis Treatment Blend" to one cup (8 oz or 250 ml) of unscented bath gel or liquid soap to create a healing bath gel.

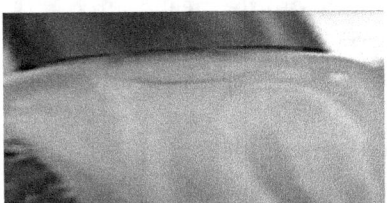

Bath Salts.

Mix 2 cups Epsom salts, 1 cup sea salt and 1 cup baking soda. Add 50 drops (2.5 ml) of the "Arthritis Treatment Blend" and a few drops of food coloring (optional). Add one cup of these bath salts to your warm bath water for a pain relieving soak.

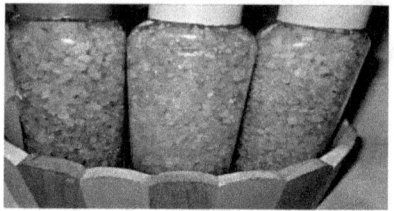

Bath Bombs.

Mix 2 oz (60 ml) of witch hazel with 20 drops of the "Arthritis Treatment Blend" in a spray bottle. Mix 2 cups baking soda, 1 cup citric acid, 1 cup sea salt, 1 cup corn starch, and 1 tablespoon olive oil in a bowl as you moisten them by spraying the witch hazel mixture. Once they start getting sticky, pack them into ice cube molds and let them dry overnight. Remove from the molds and let them air dry for two days before using them.

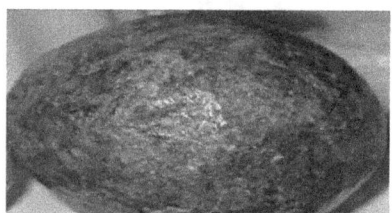

Bath Melts.

Put 2 oz. (60 grams) shea butter and 2 oz. (60 grams) cocoa butter in a glass bowl and melt them in a double boiler or in the microwave for several 10 second bursts. Once they have melted add 2 fl oz. (30 ml) of olive oil, stir with a metal spoon and remove from the heat source and let the mixture cool. Add 10 -20 drops of the "Arthritis Treatment Blend" drop by drop as you stir until you get your desired scent. Pour the mixture into ice cube trays and let it harden for several hours. Once hardened, turn the molds over to remove the bath melts.

Bath Tea.

Mix 2 cups of herbs like lavender flowers and rosemary leaves with 15 drops of the "Arthritis Treatment Blend" and 1 cup of sea salt. Put the mixture in an air tight jar or you can add a scoopful of the mixture into a cotton bath tea bag and store the filled bath tea bags in the air tight jar.

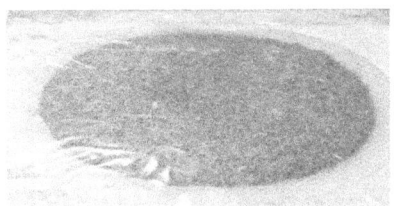

Body Wrap.

Add 20 drops of the "Arthritis Treatment Blend" to 3 oz or 100 ml of distilled water and spray it on your towel. Wrap your body in the towel and then wrap a plastic sheet around yourself and relax for 20 minutes before you unwrap yourself. This is especially beneficial for back pains.

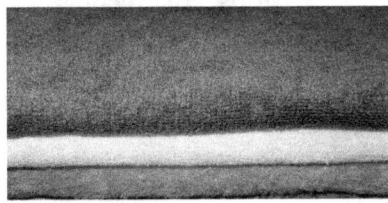

Body Compress.

Add 25 drops (1.25 ml or ¼ teaspoon) of the "Arthritis Treatment Blend" to ½ cup (4 oz or 125 ml) of warm water, dip your hand towel or bath cloth or sponge in it and wipe the aching joints with it after stepping out of the shower or bath tub.

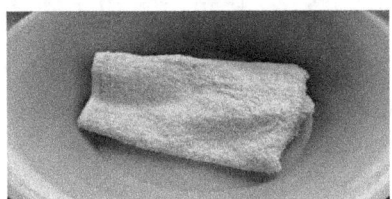

Body Oil.

Add 50 drops (2.5 ml or ½ teaspoons) of the "Arthritis Treatment Blend" to one cup (8 oz or 250 ml) of jojoba or another carrier oil and use it as an after shower body oil. Massage it into your moist skin, especially over the painful joints, to lock in the healing benefits of the essential oils.

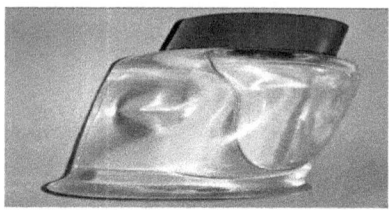

Body Butter.

Melt 1 oz. (30 grams) beeswax and 4 oz. (120 grams) pure shea butter in a double boiler or in the microwave for several 10 second bursts. Once they have melted add 3 fl oz. (90 ml) olive oil, stir and remove from the heat source. Let the mixture cool until it begins to form a cloudy layer on top. Add 10-20 drops of the "Arthritis Treatment Blend" drop by drop until you get your desired scent. Whip the mixture with a stick blender until it forms soft peaks. Spoon the whipped body butter into wide mouthed containers.

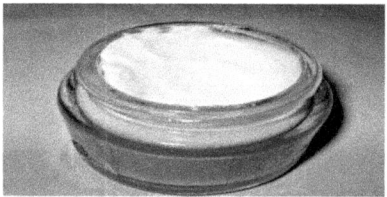

Body Lotion.

Heat 6 oz (190 ml) of sweet almond oil and 1.5 oz (45 grams) of grated beeswax in a double boiler until they mix. Remove from the heat and let the mixture cool completely. Put 8 oz (250 ml) water in a blender and with the blender on high speed, slowly pour in the cooled oil and beeswax mixture. Blend it until it emulsifies or forms a thick lotion. Add 10-20 drops of the "Arthritis Treatment Blend" drop by drop until you get your required scent. Pour the lotion in a glass jar.

Aloe Vera Aromatherapy Gel.

Add 50 drops of the "Arthritis Treatment Blend" to one cup (8 oz or 250 ml) of natural aloe vera gel to create a non-greasy, healing moisturizer.

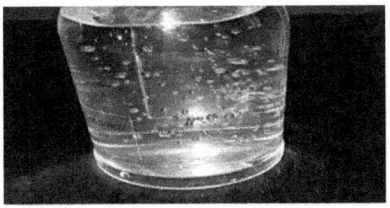

Body Massage Oil.

Add 50 drops (2.5 ml or ½ teaspoons) of the "Arthritis Treatment Blend" to one cup (8 oz or 250 ml) of jojoba or another carrier oil to create a pain relieving massage oil to massage aching joints.

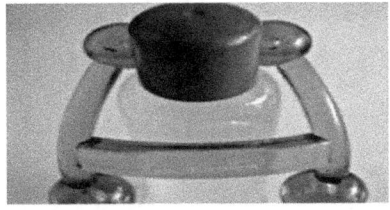

Mini Self Massage Oil.

Add 1 drop of the "Arthritis Treatment Blend" to 5 ml of jojoba or another carrier oil and put it in a small bottle that can fit into your purse to pocket. Carry it with you for 5 minute mini – self massages to massage your aching hand joints.

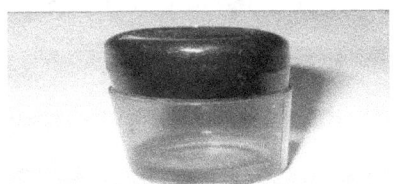

Foot Bath.

Create your own soothing foot bath blend by adding 12 drops of the "Arthritis Treatment Blend" to a bowl of warm water to soak your feet and relieve aching foot joints.

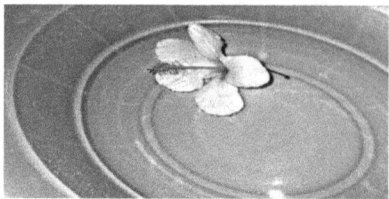

Foot Oil.

Add 6 drops the "Arthritis Treatment Blend" to 30 ml of jojoba or another carrier oil of your choice. Use it to massage your feet after your foot bath before you wrap them in soft cotton socks. You can also use it to soften your hands by massaging them and then sleeping with cotton socks.

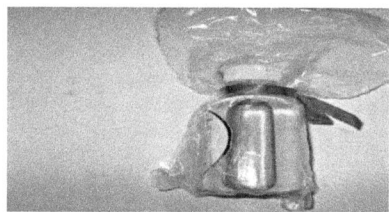

Foot Roller.

Give yourself a foot massage by applying an aromatherapy foot oil to your feet and then moving them to and fro on the foot roller. This will help ease tension and improve the circulation of blood in your feet and even reduce some types of foot pain.

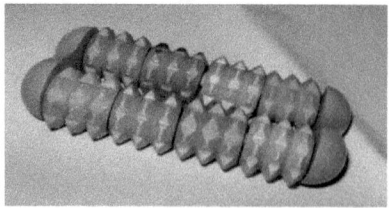

Beeswax Hand Cream.

Melt 4 tablespoons of beeswax and 2 tablespoons of shea butter. Remove from the heat source and add 8 tablespoons of sweet almond oil or any other carrier oil you may have. Mix thoroughly and when the mixture cools, add 12 drops of the "Arthritis Treatment Blend".

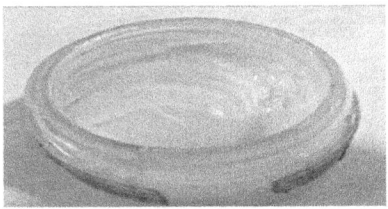

Petroleim Jelly Hand Cream.

Melt 2 teaspoons of a petroleum jelly such as Vaseline, add 6 drops of the "Arthritis Treatment Blend" when cool and then pour into a jar.

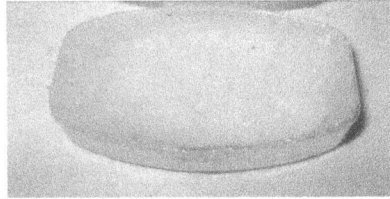

Hand Oil.

Add 6 drops the "Arthritis Treatment Blend" to 30 ml of jojoba or another carrier oil. Use it to massage your hands after washing them and then wear cotton gloves to soften them.

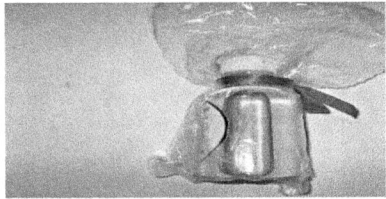

Acupressure Balls.

Give yourself a hand massage by applying the aromatherapy hand oil to your hands and then rolling these balls in the palms of your hands. This will help ease tension and improve the circulation of blood in your hands.

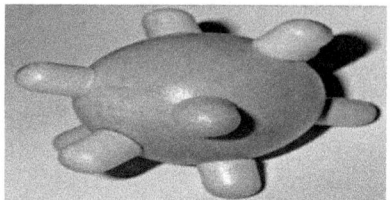

* * * * *

5

LIFESTYLE MODIFICATIONS

Lifestyle modifications that can help lower high blood pressure include:

1.

Exercise Regularly

Regular exercise is very important for managing arthritis since it:

1. Helps reduce excess body weight which contributes to joint pains

2. Helps increase joint flexibility

3. Helps increase muscle mass and strengthen muscles and tendons

Therefore aim to exercise for at least 30 minutes four days a week. If you have been leading a sedentary lifestyle, consult your doctor before making changes to your exercise regimen.

***

2.

Loose Excess Weight

Losing weight is vital for managing arthritis since the excess weight places extra pressure on the knees, hips, and ankles. In overweight and obese patients, weight loss can significantly relieve pain, most likely by reducing the stress exerted on the joint during weight bearing activities such as walking.

Before you embark on your weight loss plan, consult your nutritionist for your diet may need to be tweaked. Once you have been medically and nutritionally cleared, begin exercising by combining stretching, aerobic and weight bearing exercises.

***

3.

Manage Stress

Effective stress management is important for managing arthritis since arthritis is a chronic, painful and expensive condition that can increases stress levels.

Therefore, learn effective relaxation techniques so that you can manage stress effectively.

***

4.

Avoid High Shoes

Women are advised to avoid high-heeled shoes because they place more compressive pressures on the knees than flat or low-heeled shoes. Therefore, wear low-heeled shoes to reduce the forces that your joints and especially your knees, experience.

***

5.

Apply heat

Applying heat from heating pads, electric blankets and hot packs can reduce the pain of aching joints.

***

6.

Apply cold

Applying cold from ice cube packs or washcloths dipped in cold water can reduce the swelling and pain of inflamed joints.

***

7.

Foster Spiritual Health

Develop a strong spiritual relationship with God since several studies have shown that people of faith are healthier than non-believers. Other studies have also shown that prayer can reduce the symptoms of some diseases.

Having a relationship with your God can also help you cope with the stress and depression of living with a chronic condition like arthritis.

Therefore, find a Bible preaching Church and practice your faith sincerely since simply going through the motions does not confer any of the faith related health benefits.

* * * * *

6

EXERCISE PLAN

A balanced exercise plan should combine stretching, weight bearing and aerobic exercises.

If you have been leading a sedentary lifestyle, consult your doctor and nutritionist before making changes to your exercise regimen.

In addition, invest in a good pair of sports shoes that will cushion your feet and redistribute your weight evenly as you walk, jog, jump or run.

If as you exercise, you experience any of the following symptoms, stop exercising at once and consult your doctor: chest pain, pressure or tightness, unusual shortness of breath, pain in the jaw, arm, neck or shoulder, palpitations or skipped heart beats, feeling dizzy or fainting, muscle pain that is more severe than just discomfort.

1.

Stretching Exercises

Stretch for at least 10 minutes each morning and evening and in the warm up and cool down periods just before or right after your exercise sessions.

To stretch correctly you should:

1. Not hold your breath as you stretch. Breathe in and out rhythmically.

2. Never bounce into or out of your stretches. Gently move into and out of the various positions.

3. Hold the stretch position for 10 seconds and gradually increase the duration.

4. Be systematic and begin with the legs as you work your way up the body to the neck or vice versa.

5. Stop stretching if you feel any pain but continue if you experience mild discomfort.

The following is a list of exercises that you can do at home to stretch your entire body.

1. Neck Stretch - Stand with your feet shoulder width apart and your chin on your chest. Rotate your head once clockwise. Return chest to chin and rotate it counter clockwise. Do several rotations. Turn your face to the right, look as far back over your shoulder as you can. Hold for a count of 10. Repeat on opposite side.

2. Chest, Shoulder and Arm Stretch - Stand with your feet shoulder width apart and your knees slightly bent. Clasp your hands behind your back and push them back as far as you can reach. Push your chest forward as far as it can reach. Hold and return to starting position.

3. Side Stretch - Stand straight with your arms raised over your head. Tilt your body to the left side as you stretch your side muscles. Hold. Repeat on the opposite side.

4. Abs, Glutes and Quads Stretch - Stand with your feet together. Reach forward with your right arm. Lift your left leg behind you and grasp your left ankle with your left hand. Lift your left thigh as high as you can or until it is parallel to the ground. Repeat on opposite side.

5. Back Stretch - Lie on your back and pull both knees to your chest. Release them and lower your knees to the right side and then to the left side. Return knees back to chest.

6. Hamstring Stretch - Lie on your back with your legs bent and both feet flat on the floor. Straighten and raise your right leg. Gently pull your right thigh towards your body and hold for a count of 10. Repeat on the opposite side.

***

2.

Weight Bearing Exercises

To weight train or strength train correctly you should:

a) Not hold your breath or strain as you train.

b) Not exercise the same muscle groups for two consecutive days.

c) Aim for 3 sets of 10 repetitions each.

The following are exercises that you can do at home to strength train your entire body.

1. Overhead Press - (Works shoulders) Sit on a chair; hold a weight (or a full water bottle) in each hand at shoulder level with palms facing forward. Raise your arms straight up over your head. Lower them to shoulder level.

2. Biceps Curl - (Works biceps) Sit on a chair; hold a weight (or a full water bottle) in each hand palms facing forward. Bend your elbow and lift the weight towards your shoulder. Return to starting position and repeat with the other arm.

3. Triceps Dips - (Works triceps) Sit on the edge of a sturdy chair with your back and shoulders straight. Hold the edge of a chair and bend your elbows to form a right angle as you lower your butt off the seat to the floor. Straighten your arms and press back up to raise your butt back to the seat.

4. Push Ups - (Works deltoids, triceps, pectorals) Lie on floor, palms face down, elbows bent next to shoulders. Push up from floor by straightening elbows and contracting abs so that your body forms a straight line from your head to heel (beginners can rest both knees on floor) Lower yourself to floor by bending elbows. Push back up.

5. Simple Straight Crunches - (Works abs) Lie flat on your back; bend knees while keeping your feet flat on the floor. Place your hands on your thighs. Exhale and lift shoulder blades from the floor as you slide your hands up to your knees. Hold for a count of 10. Return to starting position and repeat.

6. Simple Side Crunches - (Works abs) Lie flat on your back; bend knees while keeping your feet flat on the floor. Place your hands on your right thigh. Exhale and lift shoulder blades from the floor as you slide your hands up to your right knee. Hold for a count of 10. Return to starting position and repeat. Do on opposite side.

7. Advanced Straight Crunches - (Works abs) Lie flat on your back; bend your knees until thighs are perpendicular to floor. Place arms crossed over your chest. Exhale, tighten abs and lift shoulder blades from the floor as you reach towards knees. Hold for a count of 10. Return to starting position and repeat.

8. Advanced Side Crunches - (Works abs) Lie flat on your back; bend your knees until thighs are perpendicular to floor. Place arms crossed over your chest. Exhale, tighten abs and lift shoulder blades from floor as you reach towards right knee. Hold for a count of 10. Return to starting position and repeat. Do on opposite side.

9. Leg Lifts - Lie on your back; legs straight; hands under butt. Lift legs 30 cm from the floor. Hold for a count of 10.

10. Lunge - (Works glutes, hamstrings, quadriceps) Stand with feet shoulder width apart, arms at sides. Take a large step forward with your left leg and ensure your left knee is above your left foot. Lower your body to the floor by bending the right knee until right thigh is parallel to the floor and right knee is close to the ground. Squeeze your glutes as you press back up to your starting position. Repeat on opposite side.

11. Squat - (Works your butt and thighs) Stand with your feet parallel and shoulder width apart. Stretch out your hands in front of you. Keeping your abs and butt tight, bend your knees and slowly lower yourself as though you are sitting. Ensure your knees don't extend past your toes. Hold for a count of 10. As your rise, squeeze your glutes.

12. Calf Raises - (Work your calf muscles) Stand with feet together and arms raised above your head. Lift your heels so that you are standing on the balls of your feet/toes. Stand on your toes for a count of 10.

***

3.

Aerobic Exercises

Aerobic exercises include walking, skipping a rope, jogging (on a treadmill or in the park), cycling or spinning in the gym, swimming, aerobic classes in a gym, sports like tennis and basketball as well as everyday activities like climbing stairs, housework and gardening.

Swimming is a good option especially if you are overweight or obese because it does not put excessive pressure on the joints of the lower limbs.

To reap the most benefits from your aerobic exercise sessions, you should:

1. Exercise for at least 30 min each session

2. Reach your Target Heart Rate (THR) which is calculated by

220 - your age = maximum heart rate (MHR)

MHR x 0.65 = minimum target heart rate (MinTHR)

MHR x 0.80 = maximum target heart rate (MaxTHR)

For example, if you are 40 years old, 220 - 40 years = 180 your maximum heart rate (MHR)

180 (MHR) x 0.65 = 117 your minimum target heart rate (MinTHR)

180 (MHR) x 0.80 = 144 your maximum target heart rate (MaxTHR)

Therefore, as you exercise, you should ensure that your heart rate is between 117 and 144.

To know your heart rate per minute, take your pulse on your wrist or neck for one minute.

The following is a rough guide of target heart rates for different age groups:

If you are 20 years old, your Target Heart Rate (THR) per minute should be 130 - 160

If you are 30 years old, your Target Heart Rate (THR) per minute should be 123 – 152

If you are 40 years old, your Target Heart Rate (THR) per minute should be 117 – 144

If you are 50 years old, your Target Heart Rate (THR) per minute should be 110 – 136

If you are 60 years old, your Target Heart Rate (THR) per minute should be 104 – 128

If you are 70 years old, your Target Heart Rate (THR) per minute should be 97 – 120

If you are 80 years old, your Target Heart Rate (THR) per minute should be 91 – 112

***

Exercise Plan

You can modify this plan to suit your lifestyle and level of activity.

Exercise Activity for Week 1

Day 1

Whole body stretch to warm up

30 min walk at minimum THR

Whole body stretch to cool down

Day 2

Whole body stretch to warm up

10 push ups, 10 triceps dips, 10 crunches

Whole body stretch to cool down

Day 3

Whole body stretch to warm up

30 min walk at minimum THR

Whole body stretch to cool down

Day 4

Whole body stretch to warm up

10 squats, 10 lunges, 10 calf raises, 10 crunches

Whole body stretch to cool down

Day 5

Whole body stretch to warm up

30 min walk at minimum THR

Whole body stretch to cool down

Exercise Activity for week 2

Day 1

Whole body stretch to warm up

30 min walk/ jog at medium THR

Whole body stretch to cool down

Day 2

Whole body stretch to warm up

15 push ups, 15 bicep curls, 15 triceps dips, 15 crunches

Whole body stretch to cool down

Day 3

Whole body stretch to warm up

30 min walk/ jog at medium THR

Whole body stretch to cool down

Day 4

Whole body stretch to warm up

15 squats, 15 lunges, 15 calf raises, 15 crunches

Whole body stretch to cool down

Day 5

Whole body stretch to warm up

30 min walk/ jog at medium THR

Whole body stretch to cool down

Exercise Activity for week 3

Day 1

Whole body stretch to warm up

30 min walk/run maximum THR

Whole body stretch to cool down

Day 2

Whole body stretch to warm up

20 push ups, 20 bicep curls, 20 triceps dips, 20 crunches

Whole body stretch to cool down

Day 3

Whole body stretch to warm up

30 min walk/run maximum THR

Whole body stretch to cool down

Day 4

Whole body stretch to warm up

20 squats, 20 lunges, 20 calf raises, 20 crunches

Whole body stretch to cool down

Day 5

Whole body stretch to warm up

30 min walk/run maximum THR

Whole body stretch to cool down

Exercise Activity for week 4

Day 1

Whole body stretch to warm up

30 min walk/run maximum THR

Whole body stretch to cool down

Day 2

Whole body stretch to warm up

30 push ups, 30 bicep curls, 30 triceps dips, 30 crunches

Whole body stretch to cool down

Day 3

Whole body stretch to warm up

30 min walk/run maximum THR

Whole body stretch to cool down

Day 4

Whole body stretch to warm up

30 push ups, 30 bicep curls, 30 triceps dips, 30 crunches

Whole body stretch to cool down

Day 5

Whole body stretch to warm up

30 min walk/run maximum THR

Whole body stretch to cool down

* * * * *

7

STRESS MANAGEMENT PLAN

Learning and practicing relaxation techniques is a very effective way of managing stress. These relaxation techniques include:

1.

Meditation

Meditation is another effective relaxation technique for coping with stress. To meditate, simply lie down in a quiet place and take several deep breaths. Once your body begins to feel calmer, focus on your inhalation and on the pure oxygen entering your body. As you exhale, envision you whole body relaxing. You can also meditate on Scriptures like **With God all things are possible** (Matthew 19:26) and envisioning your stressful situation resolving miraculously.

***

2.

Abdominal Breathing

Abdominal breathing or deep breathing is one fastest ways of counteracting the body's stress response. It is done by inhaling through your nose until your abdomen rises, holding your breath for a few moments and then exhaling completely through your mouth until your abdomen collapses. This cycle of filling the lungs with air, pausing and then emptying them can be repeated for 15 minutes every day.

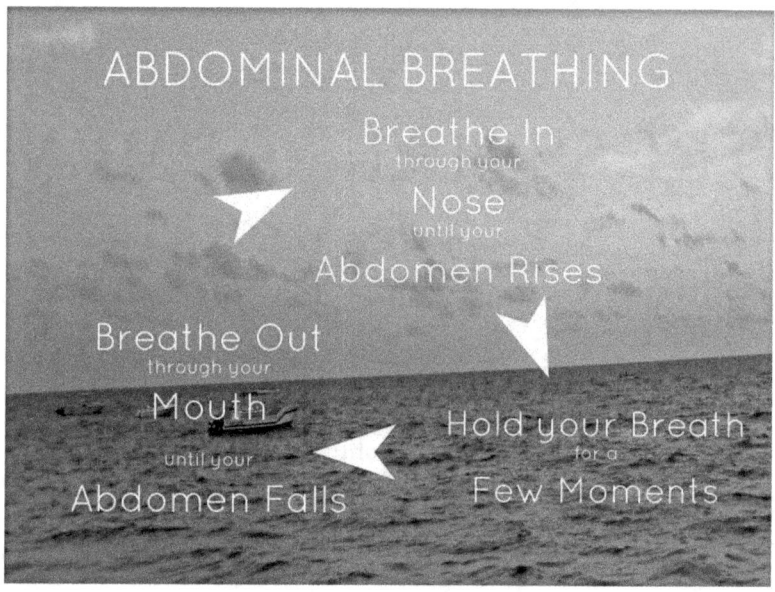

***

3.

Guided Imagery

Guided imagery is another effective relaxation technique. It involves visualizing yourself in a relaxing environment. Therefore close your eyes, take several deep breaths and use your mind's eye to see yourself relaxing on a beach or floating on a cloud or walking through a garden or whichever environment makes you feel relaxed. Use all your senses to immerse yourself in the restful environment by seeing soothing images, smelling appealing scents, hearing calming sounds, tasting and feeling your way through it. After you have enjoyed our visit, bring yourself gently back to reality.

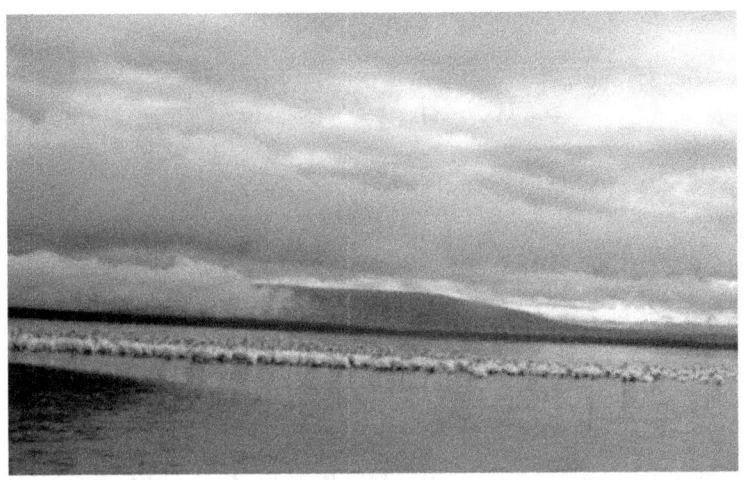

***

4.

Problem Solving Visualization

Visualization can also be used to manage stressful situations. To do this see yourself with your mind's eye in your most stressful situation and then envisioning yourself using various strategies to cope. For example you can imagine yourself dealing with a stressful boss by breathing deeply until you no longer feel distressed by their words or actions.

***

5.

Physical Exercise

When a person is stressed, they tense their muscles. Stretching exercises reduce this muscle tension and help a person feel relaxed.

Aerobic exercises help the body burn circulating stress hormones that contribute to the development of stress related illnesses.

Weight bearing exercises also aid in stress management since they demand concentration and help a person forget their problems.

Therefore engage in regular physical exercises to manage stress.

***

Relaxing Activities

Other relaxing activities that you can engage in to manage stress include:

1. Journaling since writing down uncensored feelings is a very effective method of catharsis. It is doubly effective when combined with writing lists of things you are thankful for.

2. Listening to calming music.

3. Engaging in hobbies that complement their main job

4. Helping less fortunate members of your society like visiting the sick in hospitals since this takes your mind off your problems

5. Drinking soothing herbal teas like chamomile and passionflower.

6. Eating foods which raise serotonin levels like turkey, salmon, chicken, cheese, chocolate, wholegrain bread.

7. Watching comedy since laughter relieves tension.

8. Spending time with your social support system.

***

Stress Management Plan

Stress Management Plan Week 1

Day 1

1. Abdominal breathing

2. Meditation

3. Physical Exercise

4. Watching Comedy

Day 2

1. Abdominal breathing

2. Meditation

3. Drinking herbal teas and eating serotonin rich foods

4. Watching Comedy

Day 3

1. Abdominal breathing

2. Meditation

3. Physical Exercise

4. Watching Comedy

Day 4

1. Abdominal breathing

2. Meditation

3. Drinking herbal teas and eating serotonin rich foods

4. Watching Comedy

Day 5

1. Abdominal breathing

2. Meditation

3. Physical Exercise

4. Watching Comedy

Day 6 and 7

1. Abdominal breathing 2. Meditation 3. Spending time with your social support system

Stress Management Plan Week 2

Day 1

1. Abdominal breathing

2. Guided imagery

3. Physical Exercise

4. Listening to Music

Day 2

1. Abdominal breathing

2. Guided imagery

3. Drinking herbal teas and eating serotonin rich foods

4. Listening to Music

Day 3

1. Abdominal breathing

2. Guided imagery

3. Physical Exercise

4. Listening to Music

Day 4

1. Abdominal breathing

2. Guided imagery

3. Drinking herbal teas and eating serotonin rich foods

4. Listening to Music

Day 5

1. Abdominal breathing

2. Guided imagery

3. Physical Exercise

4. Listening to Music

Day 6 and 7

1. Abdominal breathing 2. Guided imagery 3. Engaging in Complementary Hobbies

Stress Management Plan Week 3

Day 1

1. Abdominal breathing

2. Problem solving visualization

3. Physical Exercise

4. Journaling and writing gratitude lists

Day 2

1. Abdominal breathing

2. Problem solving visualization

3. Drinking herbal teas and eating serotonin rich foods

4. Journaling and writing gratitude lists

Day 3

1. Abdominal breathing

2. Problem Solving Visualization

3. Physical Exercise

4. Journaling and writing gratitude lists

Day 4

1. Abdominal breathing

2. Problem Solving Visualization

3. Drinking herbal teas and eating serotonin rich foods

4. Journaling and writing gratitude lists

Day 5

1. Abdominal breathing

2. Problem Solving Visualization

3. Physical Exercise

4. Journaling and writing gratitude lists

Day 6 and 7

1. Abdominal breathing 2. Problem Solving Visualization 3. Helping the less fortunate

Stress Management Plan Week 4

Day 1

1. Abdominal breathing

2. Meditation or Guided Imagery or Problem Solving Visualization (choose the one that has been most relaxing for you and practice it regularly)

3. Physical exercise

4. Watching Comedy or Listening to Music or Journaling and writing gratitude lists (choose the one that has been most relaxing for you and practice it regularly)

Day 2

1. Abdominal breathing

2. Meditation or Guided Imagery or Problem Solving Visualization (choose the one that has been most relaxing for you and practice it regularly)

3. Drinking herbal teas and eating serotonin rich foods

4. Watching Comedy or Listening to Music or Journaling and writing gratitude lists (choose the one that has been most relaxing for you and practice it regularly)

Day 3

1. Abdominal breathing

2. Meditation or Guided Imagery or Problem Solving Visualization (choose the one that has been most relaxing for you and practice it regularly)

3. Physical exercise

4. Watching Comedy or Listening to Music or Journaling and writing gratitude lists (choose the one that has been most relaxing for you and practice it regularly)

Day 4

1. Abdominal breathing

2. Meditation or Guided Imagery or Problem Solving Visualization (choose the one that has been most relaxing for you and practice it regularly)

3. Drinking herbal teas and eating serotonin rich foods

4. Watching Comedy or Listening to Music or Journaling and writing gratitude lists (choose the one that has been most relaxing for you and practice it regularly)

Day 5

1. Abdominal breathing

2. Meditation or Guided Imagery or Problem Solving Visualization (choose the one that has been most relaxing for you and practice it regularly)

3. Physical exercise

4. Watching Comedy or Listening to Music or Journaling and writing gratitude lists (choose the one that has been most relaxing for you and practice it regularly)

Day 6 and 7

1. Abdominal breathing

2. Meditation or Guided Imagery or Problem Solving Visualization (choose the one that has been most relaxing for you and practice it regularly)

3. Spending time with your social support system or Engaging in complementary hobbies or Helping the less fortunate (choose the one that has been most relaxing for you and practice it regularly)

###

ABOUT THE AUTHOR

Dr. Miriam Kinai is a medical doctor and freelance health writer/blogger.

You can visit her blog at http://www.MyBlogBookClub.com or follow her on twitter at http://twitter.com/AlmasiHealth

Email enquiries to almasihealthcare@yahoo.com with BOOKS as your subject.

HERBS AND SPICES FOR THE COOK, HEALER AND BEAUTICIAN

Herbs and Spices for the Cook, Healer and Beautician uses color pictures and clear explanations to teach you about more than 70 healing herbs and spices.

You will learn about their:

* Therapeutic (healing) uses

* Drug interactions

* Contraindications (when not to use them)

* Cooking tips

* Beauty tips

*****

INTERNATIONAL GOURMET HERB AND SPICE BLENDS

International Gourmet Herb and Spice Blends teaches you how to prepare exotic herb and spice blends from around the world. You will discover the recipes for:

* Barbecue Rub, Cajun, Apple Pie and Pumpkin Pie Spice Mixes from America

* Pudding Spice Mix from Britain

* 5 Spice Mix from China

* Berbere Spice Mix from Ethiopia

* Curry Powder and Garam Masala from India

* Bouquet Garni, Herbs de Provence and Quatre Epices from France

* Herb Mix from Italy

* Jerk Seasoning from Jamaica

* Shichimi Togarashi from Japan

* Pilau Spice Blend from Kenya

* Chili Powder from Mexico

* Baharat Spice Blend from the Middle East

* Ras El Hanout from Morocco

*****

THE QUICK GOURMET CHEF

The Quick Gourmet is an essential culinary skills cookbook which teaches how to make simple, divine dishes.

You will learn how to make:

* Hot Chocolate Mixes and Drinks

* Hot Chai Tea Mixes and Drinks

* Hot Coffee Mixes and Drinks

* Sensational Smoothies

* Non-Dairy Smoothies

* Chocolate Covered Strawberries

* Chocolate Truffles

* Healthy Chicken Salads

* Healthy Tuna Salads

* Savory Salsas

* Herb Butter

* Cheese Dips and Sauces

* Gourmet Sandwiches

* Perfect Hard Boiled Eggs

* A Cheese Board

* Natural Food Color

*****

HOW TO STYLE AND PHOTOGRAPH FOOD

Regardless of whether you are an aspiring food blogger or you want to make money online selling stock photos, How To Style and Photograph Food, uses color pictures and clear explanations to teach you the food photography tips that can help you improve your digital camera photography skills so that you can begin photographing food like a pro.

You will learn:

* The equipment that you need

* How to set up the lighting

* How to prepare the stage

* How to style the food

* How to shoot the food

*****

HOW TO MAKE NATURAL SKIN CARE PRODUCTS VOLUME 1

How To Make Natural Skin Care Products Volume 1 by Dr Miriam Kinai is filled with recipes for making organic bath and body products for normal, sensitive, oily and dry skin types as well as therapeutic products to manage mature skin, prematurely aging skin, cellulite, eczema, psoriasis, ringworms, dandruff, thinning hair, menopausal symptoms, pre-menstrual tension (PMS), painful periods, arthritis, stress, sadness or depression, mental exhaustion and insomnia.

This book also teaches you the best vegetable oils, essential oils, natural butters and herbs to use when making products for different skin types physical conditions. You will learn how to make:

* Bath bombs

* Bath melts

* Bath salts

* Bath teas

* Body butters

* Body lotions

* Body scrubs

* Healing balms and body creams

* Herb infused oils

* Natural soap

How to Make Natural Skin Care Products Volume 1 will leave you with a clear understanding of how to make bath and beauty products to use in your home or to give as gifts or to sell and make money.

*****

ORGANIC SKIN CARE PRODUCT INGREDIENTS

Organic Skin Care Product Ingredients teaches you about the different natural substances that can be used to create natural bath and beauty products to use in your home or to give as gifts to your loved ones or to sell and make money.

You will learn about:

* Natural butters

* Natural clays

* Natural colorants

* Natural exfoliants

* Natural fragrances

* Natural oils

* Natural preservatives

*****

THE ESSENTIALS OF AROMATHERAPY ESSENTIAL OILS

The Essentials of Aromatherapy Essential Oils by Dr Miriam Kinai teaches you how to use aromatherapy oils to improve your physical, mental and emotional well being.

The author's experience as a medical doctor and clinical aromatherapy practitioner have enabled her to write a highly informative guide for those who want to utilize the healing benefits of these natural plant essences.

You will discover:

* The safety information and therapeutic uses of 18 essential oils

* How to blend essential oils

* The characteristics and uses of 14 carrier oils

* How to Dilute Essential Oils with Carrier Oils

* How to Use Essential Oils

* Cautionary Measures when using Essential Oils

* Numerous Essential Oil Recipes for bath products as well as skin care and hair care products

The Essentials of Aromatherapy Essential Oils will leave you with a clear understanding of how you can safely use aromatherapy essential oils to heal yourself naturally.

*****

CARRIER OILS GUIDE

Carrier Oils Guide teaches you the characteristics, health benefits and uses of commonly used carrier oils. You will learn about:

* Apricot Kernel Oil

* Avocado Oil

* Borage Seed Oil

* Calendula Oil

* Carrot Seed Oil

* Castor Oil

* Evening Primrose Oil

* Fractionated Coconut Oil

* Jojoba

* Olive Oil

* Rosehip Oil

* Sunflower Oil

* Sweet Almond Oil

* Virgin Coconut Oil

* Useful formulas for Diluting Essential Oils with Carrier Oils

*****

MEDICAL AROMATHERAPY FOR HEALTH PROFESSIONALS

Medical Aromatherapy for Healthcare Professionals by Dr Miriam Kinai teaches you how to use essential oils to treat physical diseases and emotional disorders.

The author's experience as a medical doctor and clinical aromatherapy practitioner have enabled her to write a highly informative guide for those who want to utilize the healing benefits of these natural plant essences.

You will discover how to use essential oils to:

* Treat skin diseases like acne, eczema and psoriasis

* Treat other physical diseases like high blood pressure, arthritis, coughs and colds

* Manage mental and emotional conditions like anxiety, depression, anger and stress

* Relieve the symptoms of menopause and premenstrual tension

* Lessen insomnia and impotence

Medical Aromatherapy for Healthcare Professionals is therefore an essential resource for holistic healthcare practitioners like massage therapists, naturopaths and herbalists.

It is also a useful resource for conventional medicine healthcare providers like physicians and nurses who want to begin practicing integrative medicine and for patients who want to improve their health naturally by using aromatherapy oils.

*****

AROMATHERAPY COURSE

Aromatherapy Course by Dr Miriam Kinai tutors you on how to use essential oils to improve your physical, mental and emotional well being.

The author's experience as a medical doctor and clinical aromatherapy practitioner have enabled her to create a highly informative course on how to use these natural plant essences.

You will learn:

* The safety information and therapeutic uses of essential oils like clary sage, eucalyptus, geranium, grapefruit, lavender, lemon, lemongrass, marjoram, orange (sweet), patchouli, peppermint, Roman chamomile, rose, rosemary, sandalwood, spearmint, tea tree and ylang ylang.

* The safety information and therapeutic uses of carrier oils like apricot kernel oil, avocado oil, borage seed oil, calendula oil, carrot seed oil, castor oil, evening primrose oil, fractionated coconut oil, jojoba, olive oil, rosehip oil, sunflower oil, sweet almond oil and virgin coconut oil.

* How to blend essential oils

* How to dilute essential oils with carrier oils

* How to administer essential oils

* How to make natural healing products from numerous aromatherapy recipes

* How to utilize the healing benefits of essentials oils even if you do not have prior training in aromatherapy

The Aromatherapy Course will leave you with a clear understanding of how you can heal yourself and your family naturally by using essentials oils on your body and in your home.

*****

DEALING WITH DEPRESSION NATURALLY

Dealing with Depression Naturally presents a holistic approach to managing depression with natural antidepressants. You will learn how to treat depression with:

* Aromatherapy

* Art therapy

* Christian Biblical principles

* Chromotherapy

* Diet therapy

* Eco-therapy

* Herbal therapy

* Home decor therapy

* Music therapy

* Phototherapy

* Exercise therapy

* Self-Psychotherapy

* Social therapy

* Talk therapy

* Vitamin therapy

* Writing therapy

*****

CHRISTIAN LIFE COACHING HANDBOOK

Christian Life Coaching Handbook offers a Biblical approach to managing different aspects of life.

You will learn:

* Christian anger management

* Christian conflict resolution

* Christian depression treatment

* Christian goal setting

* Christian marital stress management

* Christian stress management

* How to assert yourself

* How to defeat fear

* How to love yourself

* How to overcome shyness

* How to resist temptation

* How to stop being a people pleaser

*****

CHRISTIAN PERSONAL FINANCE

Christian Personal Finance teaches Biblical principles of money management.

You will learn:

* Christian financial stress management from people who were dealing with money stress like the Acts 3 beggar or credit issues like the widow in second Kings.

* Biblical prosperity principles from wealthy men and women of God like Isaac and the Proverbs 31 woman.

* Bible verses to use as spiritual warfare prayers and as Christian finance affirmations and Christian money meditations.

*****

ANTHOLOGY OF CHRISTIAN BIBLE SERMONS

Anthology of Christian Bible Sermons is a compilation of more than 20 Biblical rhema teachings which include:

* A New Christmas Message

* A New Easter Message

* Are You A Flamboyant Fig Tree Christian?

* Biblical Lessons for Purim from Queen Esther

* Can God Help Me If I Am Surrounded By Enemies?

* How Badly Do You Really Want It?

* Seed Words And The Powerful Tongue

* Spiritual AIDS

* The Three Levels Of Getting Lost

* Why Does God Allow Suffering?

* Your Life Is Your Ministry And Your Storm Is Your Message

* A Perfect God, Imperfect People, and Perfect Plans

* We Are Not Ignorant of His Devices

* How to Prepare for a Dangerous Journey

* Yes, God Can

* How to Serve the Body of Christ

* Conduits of God

* Go Back? Stand Still? Move Forward? Drown?

*****

CHRISTIAN SPIRITUAL WARFARE

Christian Spiritual Warfare teaches you the awesome Bible verses you can use as spiritual warfare prayers, Christian affirmations and in your Christian meditation sessions as you fight your spiritual battles.

You will learn how to fight for the following with Bible verses:

* Marriage * Children * Health

* Christian Faith * Christian Ministry

* Country

* Finances * Job * Business

* Peace of Mind * Restoration * Self Esteem * Self Love

You will also learn how to fight against the following with Bible verses:

* Addiction * Temptation

* Being Single * Infertility

* Opposition * Oppression

* Worry * Fear

* Feelings of Condemnation * Confusion

* Danger * Death * Despair * Discouragement

* Impatience * Insomnia * Laziness * Loneliness

* Poverty * Pride * Sadness

* Vengeance * Weakness

* A Foul Mouth * Lying

*****

DARK SKIN DERMATOLOGY COLOR ATLAS

Dark Skin Dermatology Color Atlas is filled with clear explanations and color photos of skin, hair, and nail diseases affecting people with skin of color or Fitzpatrick skin types IV, V, and VI.

Topics covered include Acne Vulgaris, Alopecia Areata, Anal Warts, Angioedema, Aphthous Ulcers, Atopic Dermatitis, Blastomycosis, Blister Beetle Dermatitis or Nairobi Fly Dermatitis, Cellulitis, Chronic Ulcers, Confetti Hypopigmentation, Cutaneous T Cell Lymphoma, Cutaneous Tuberculosis, Dermatitis Artefacta, Erythema Nodosum,

Exfoliative Erythroderma, Gianotti Crosti Syndrome, Hand Dermatitis, Hemangioma, Herpes Zoster, Ichthyosis, Ingrown Toenails, Irritant Contact Dermatitis, Kaposi Sarcoma, Keloids, Keratoderma Blenorrhagica, Klippel Trenaunay Weber Syndrome, Leishmaniasis, Leprosy, Leukonychia, Lichen Nitidus, Lichen Planus,

Lichenoid Drug Eruption, Linear Epidermal Nevus, Linear IgA Dermatosis (LAD), Lipodermatosclerosis, Lymphangioma Circumscriptum, Miliaria, Molluscum Contagiosum, Neurofibromatosis, Nickel Dermatitis, Onychomadesis, Onychomycosis, Palmoplantar Eccrine Hidradenitis, Papular Pruritic Eruption (PPE), Paronychia, Pellagra, Pemphigus Foliaceous,

Pemphigus Vulgaris, Piebaldism, Pityriasis Rosea, Pityriasis Rubra Pilaris, Plantar Hyperkeratosis, Plantar Warts, Poikiloderma, Postinflammatory Hyperpigmentation and Hypopigmentation, Post Topical Steroids Hypopigmentation, Psoriasis, Pyogenic Granuloma or Lobular Capillary Hemangioma, Scabies, Seborrheic Dermatitis, Steven Johnson Syndrome (SJS) and Toxic Epidermal Necrolysis (TEN),

Sunburn, Systemic Sclerosis, Tinea Capitis, Tinea Pedis, Tinea Versicolor, Traction Alopecia, Urticaria, Vasculitis, Vitiligo, and Xanthelasma.

*****

www.ingramcontent.com/pod-product-compliance
Lightning Source LLC
Chambersburg PA
CBHW070609290526
45790CB00002B/842